YOUR PARENT, MY PATIENT

The Caregiver's Perception

Dr. Latonya D. Hughes, PhD, RN

Copyright © 2019 by Latonya D. Hughes

All rights reserved. No part of this book may be reproduced or used in any manner without written permission of the copyright owner except for the use of quotations in a book review.

FIRST EDITION

ACKNOWLEDGMENTS

I am grateful to God, for He pushed me in completing this scholarly passage. To my husband Bernard and my daughter Nara thank you for the continuous support throughout this journey, I could not have achieved this without your understanding and patience. I would also like to thank my Christian friends who prayed and encouraged me when I felt as if this endeavor would not come to pass.

DEDICATION

This book is dedicated to the Nurses and CNA's working in long-term care facilities and to residents/families who all desire person-centered care.

TABLE OF CONTENTS

LIST OF TABLES ii

CHAPTERS

THE APPROACH 1

THE PROBLEM 15

THE DICUSSIONS 45

THE PERCEPTION 60

THE INTERPRETATION 73

THE IMPACT 80

REFERENCES 82

APPENDIXES

Appendix A: Invitation to Participate 101

Appendix B: Focus Group Discussion Script 102

LIST OF TABLES

Table 1. Literature Search	44
Table 2. Characteristics of the Research Participants	47
Table 3. Percentage of Theme Content	51
Table 4. Codes and References	52
Table 5. Theoretical Theme Content	53
Table 6. The Care Residents Received Word Query	54
Table 7. The Understanding of PCC Word Query	56
Table 8. PCC Word Query	57
Table 9. Theme Content per Participant Category	57
Table 10. Research Questions and Interview Questions	61
Table 11. The nurse perception of PCC	62
Table 12. A description A Caring Approach.	64
Table 13. The nurse description of PCC.	66
Table 14. The CNA's description of PCC	68
Table 15. Understanding of PCC	70
Table 16. Knowledge of PCC Provided	71

Chapter One

THE APPROACH

The long-term care industry is currently transitioning from institutional care to a more individualized care philosophy. This national movement known as patient-centered care, resident-centered care, or person-centered care, focuses on the person who is receiving care in making decisions regarding their care (Chenoweth et al., 2015; Røen et al., 2017). For purposes of this study I will refer to this change in culture as person-centered care.

Since 2008, researchers have noted that person-centered care leads to improved outcomes for the resident and caregiver Grosch, Medvene, & Wolcott, 2008; Linzer et al., 2015; Rossi et al., 2015). The general problem is we really do not know nurses' and CNAs' thoughts of person-centered care (Kusmaul & Waldrop, 2015). This research gap limits knowledge about the individualized care these caregivers are providing. This understanding could contribute to the impact on the delivery of person-centered care in long-term care settings. The residents' view of care received in long-term care facilities is well researched (Alharbi et al., 2014a; Bramley & Matiti, 2014; Ulin, Olsso

Wolf, & Ekman, 2016). However, future work is needed to better understand the perspective of the staff (Donnelly & MacEntee, 2016). Person-centered care should be made pertinent to members of the interdisciplinary team, not just the resident (Tobiano, Bucknall, Marshall, Guinane, & Chaboyer, 2015). The interdisciplinary team may have different opinions about person-centered care. More primary research involving several members of the team, rather than a single professional discipline is needed ((Tobiano et al., 2015). A closer review of nursing staff effects on individualized care in different types of healthcare settings is also needed (Bachnick, Ausserhofer, Baernholdt, Simon, & Match RN Study Group, 2018). The contribution of this study may have a potential social implication of impacting the delivery of care within long-term care settings. The major segments of this chapter include the background, the problem, the purpose of the study, the research questions, the nature of the study, definitions, assumptions, the scope and delimitations, limitations, significance, and a summary.

Background

Over the last decade, long-term care facilities have transitioned from institutional care models to models that focus on person-centered care, in which the resident is the center of the care (Andrew & Ritchie, 2017; Flagg, 2015; Van Haitsma et al., 2014). This well-researched topic supports documented efforts of the frontline staff that has provided daily care and have built relationships with the residents (McGilton, Boscart, Brown, & Bowers, 2014). The residents' life becomes more fulfilled as their desires and wishes are recognized and honored. The core elements of resident participation, relationships of residents and staff, and the context in which care is being delivered are instrumental in the successful implementation of person-centered care (Tobiano et al., 2015). Researchers have noted that person-centered care leads to improved outcomes for the resident and caregiver (Linzer et al., 2015; Rossi et al., 2015). The general problem is that nurse and CNA opinions regarding person-centered care are unknown (Kusmaul & Waldrop, 2015). The CNA provides 80% of the direct care in nursing home settings (Gray et al., 2016; Davila et al., 2016). These individuals presume to know more about the residents' desires, than other caregiver (Davila et al., 2016). However, research on the CNA and nurse perception of person-center care is limited (Chatchumni, Namvongprom, Sandborgh, Mazaheri, & Eriksson, 2015; Kusmaul & Waldrop, 2015). Although scarce, research findings suggest that organizations who are knowledgeable of the nurses' perception are more likely to limit barriers that hinder care delivery (Rodríguez-Martín, Stolt, Katajisto, & Suhonen 2015; Wilberforce et al., 2016).

This research gap limits knowledge about the individualized care these caregivers are providing. This understanding may contribute to the impact on the delivery of person-centered care in long-term care settings. The residents' view of care received in long-term care facilities is well researched (Alharbi et al., 2014; Bramley & Matiti, 2014; Ulin et al., 2016). Donnelly and MacEntee (2016) suggested that a gap in the literature exists and suggest further research is needed to understand person-centered care from the perspective of the staff.

Problem Statement

The problem is that research on the nurse and CNA opinions of person-centered care are limited (Kusmaul & Waldrop, 2015; Wilberforce et al., 2016). When the personal care worker understands the residents' unique needs, person-centered care leads to improved outcomes for the resident and the caregivers (Desmond et al., 2014; Linzer et al., 2015; Rossi et al., 2015). The residents' quality of life is improved. Barriers that hinder care delivery are limited for the caregivers (Rodríguez-Martín et al., 2015). According to Tayab and Narushima (2014), customizing the residents' preferences includes understanding their lifestyles and beliefs. The residents' perception of the caring feelings of the nursing staff has a direct association with the residents' satisfaction and healing (Keeley, Wolf, Regul, & Jadwin, 2015).

The long-term care industry is currently transitioning from institutional care to a more individualized care philosophy. This national movement known as resident centered care, resident-centered care, or person-centered care, is focused primarily on involving the resident in making decisions regarding their care (Chenoweth et al., 2015; Røen et al., 2017). For purposes of this study we will refer to this change in culture as person-centered care.

In 2017, the Center for Medicare and Medicaid Services (CMS) introduced a new regulation for long-term care organizations to provide person-centered care to all residents admitted to the long-term care and post-acute rehabilitation facilities (United States Department of Health and Human Services, 2017). The mandate required that person-centered care services were to begin within the first 48 hours of admission, as evidence by the development of a baseline plan of care.

Person-centered care services to be implemented includes the identification of the residents' goals and preferences that assist in attaining or maintaining their highest level of well-being. The baseline care plan would then be followed by a comprehensive plan of care. The comprehensive plan of care must be completed within the first 7 days of admission. At that time the resident would be given an opportunity to provide detailed information on regarding their needs, strengths, life history, personal and cultural preferences. The resident would also be given the opportunity to participate in care plan development as well as to express their preferences and potential for future discharge and return to the community (United States Department of Health and Human Services, 2017).

Researchers have noted that person-centered care leads to improved outcomes for the resident and caregiver (Linzer et al., 2015; Rossi et al., 2015). The CNA, the primary care giver for nursing home residents, is responsible for providing 80% of the care given to the nursing home residents (Gray et al., 2016). Although this topic has been researched within several healthcare settings (Abbott, Heid, & Van Haitsma, 2016; Wilberforce et al., 2016), the current literature on the perception of the caregiver, specifically the CNA is limited.

Purpose of the Study

Research on the CNA and nurse perception of person-center care is limited (Kusmaul & Waldrop, 2015; Wilberforce et al., 2016). The purpose of this study is to explore the nurses' and CNA's perception of the person-centered care services they deliver. The study will address the research gap through a qualitative approach with focused group discussions. Focus group discussions will provide opportunity for the participants to clarify and share their individual perspectives (Cleary, Horsfall, & Hayter, 2014). This design is effective in collecting data that examines knowledge and ideas, whereas Individual interviews are more appropriate for obtaining biography information (Cleary et al., 2014). The group discussions could also encourage participation of individuals who may be uncomfortable with one-on-one discussion (Cleary et al., 2014; Rauf, Baig, Jaffery, & Shafi, 2014). These persons may become engaged in group discussion generated by another group member. The research participants will include nurses (RN's and LPNs) and CNAs currently working in the same nursing home located in Chesapeake, Virginia. Two focus group discussions (one group of CNA's and one group of nurse's) will take place in the facility's conference room. The

Chesapeake facility is one of a select few facilities in the state of Virginia that offer care in an innovative household model. Hot meals are readily available 24 hours a day, 7 days per week. The household model also offers an intimate living environment that includes features such as private bedrooms, landscaped courtyards, living rooms with fireplaces and private spaces for residents and families to enjoy. These group discussions will explore the perception of the person-centered care.

Research Questions

Research Question 1

What is the nurses' and CNA's perception of person-centered care?

Research Question 2

What are the carative factors that influence the nurse and CNA's perception of person-centered care?

Theoretical Foundation

Watson's caring theory is the theoretical framework to be used for this study (Flagg, 2015). The origin of Watson's theory is centered on how the science of nursing involves a holistic approach which encompasses tuning into one's values and willingness to be committed to caring for others. Watson described caring as response to a condition; a condition of health and wellness. Watson further explained that the nurses' response was characterized by transpersonal caring relationships, caring moments, and 10 carative factors (Edvardsson, Watt, & Pearce, 2017) that include (a) humanistic altruistic system of values, (b) faith-hope, (c) sensitivity to one's self and to others, (d) helping-trust relationship, (e) positive and negative feelings, (f) creative problem-solving method for decision making, (g) interpersonal teaching-learning, (h) mental and physical, (i) sociocultural and spiritual environment, (j) gratification of human needs, and (k) phenomenological forces (Turkel, Watson, & Giovannoni, 2018). These elements offer caregivers a guide to providing person-centered care. Research on the theory of caring, gives nurses the opportunity to use Watson's ten carative factors to enhance communication, which ultimately leads to the effectiveness of professional nursing practice (Brewer & Watson, 2015). Jean Watson's theory of human caring emphasis experiences and processes associated with human caring. The theory supports caring behaviors illustrated by caregivers improve resident and nurse outcome. The residents are more satisfied with the care received and the caregivers are more satisfied with the care provided (Sitzman & Watson, 2018).

The rationale for choosing Jean Watson's theory is directly related to the theory focusing on the human caring experiences (Sitzman & Watson, 2018) and person-centered care is being characterized as a caring feeling (Bramley & Matiti, 2014; Tobiano et al., 2015). Organizations have moved from the practice of providing the nursing staff with scripts when communicating with residents and families (Cleary et al., 2014) to allowing the staff to communicate openly. The caring factor demonstrated by nursing staff has been instrumental in the culture change of an environment based on human caring (Brewer & Watson, 2015). The residents' experienced with human caring revealed that communication and responsiveness to their individual needs left them with a perception that the staff cared more. These feelings were unswervingly correlated to trust and dignity.

Watson's primary writing defines caring as human, attentive and intentional (Watson & Smith, 2002). The caregiver that is intentional is aware of the actions that are implemented. When the nurse is intentional in caring for the resident, a caring relationship between the resident and the nurse is established (Turkel et al., 2018).

The nurse and the resident becomes comfortable with one another, leaving any unknown feelings. The caregivers' choices and actions are formulated through identifying their own intentions (Bell, Campbell, & Goldberg, 2015; Watson & Brewer, 2015).

Person-centered care allows the residents desires and preferences to be brought back into care decisions. Residents have verbalized that it matters to them to have personalized services that are caring (Aiken, Rafferty & Sermeus, 2014; Edvardson et al., 2017). Caring from the resident's perspective is associated with physical and mental satisfaction (Edvardsson et al., 2017). Utilizing the carative factors of Watson's theory, the fundamental concept of caring has been associated with person-centered care and quality (Edvardsson, 2015). Caring is a science that involves experiences of providing an emotion that improve outcomes (Sitzman & Watson, 2014). The science of caring guides the caregivers in understanding what the resident perceives as caring, which in turn guides the caregiver to use caring intentionality (Drake, 2016) from the focus group sessions. The data was retrieved through an open-ended questioning format (Creswell & Creswell, 2017).

Definitions

The following section of this study provides concise definitions of key concepts and terms used in this dissertation. Terms used in the study with multiple meanings will be defined. Citations supporting the definitions have also been identified.

Carative factors: describes the ten aspects of Watson's Theory of Human Caring used to guide clinical implementation. The ten factors include: Humanistic altruistic system of values, Faith-hope, Sensitivity to one's self and to others, Helping-trust relationship, Positive and negative feelings, Creative problem-solving method for creative decision making, Interpersonal teaching-learning, Mental, physical, sociocultural, and spiritual environment, Gratification of human needs, and Phenomenological forces (Turkel et al., 2018; Watson & Brewer, 2015).

Patient-centered: describes the process of providing care that is specific to the patient's needs, values, and expressed preferences (Van Haitsma et al., 2014).

Person-centered: describes the process of both patients and health professionals forming a partnership in care delivery (Alharbi et al., 2014a; United States Department of Health and Human Services, 2017).

Perceptions: describes a person's subjective thought of an experience (Wilberforce et al., 2016).

Individualized care: describes the process of meeting the needs and preferences of a patient and considering the patient's beliefs, values, hopes, needs and desires (Wilberforce et al., 2016).

Significance

The general problem is that the nurses' and CNAs' thoughts or perceptions of person-centered care are limited (Kusmaul & Waldrop, 2015; Wilberforce et al., 2016). The study could address the research gap by exploring the nurses' and CNA's thoughts of the person-centered care services they deliver. When person-centered care is provided, the residents' quality of life is improved and barriers that hinder care delivery are limited for the caregivers (Rodríguez-Martín et al., 2015). This study may potentially contribute to the advance knowledge of nursing, as the findings may provide a better understanding of how person-centered care is perceived by the caregiver. Knowing the caregivers' perception may offer an explanation of the caring factors used in ensuring person-centered care is delivered. The caregiver may provide education to the resident and family on how to person-centered care may be provided, even when preferences maybe seen unreasonable. This study may potentially contribute to the advancement of nursing practice. When the nurse and CNA perception of person-centered care is obtained, the findings may provide a foundation for continued development in providing residents with the care they prefer. Providing care as preferred by the resident may improve the resident's quality of life, as the resident will be receiving care based on their preference. This study may potentially impact social change. When the nurse and CNA perception of person-centered care is identified, the caregiver may encourage the resident to express their individual preferences to ensure person-centered care can be provided. The clear communication may enhance the relationship with the resident and the caregiver potentially leading to systemic change in the delivery of care in long-term facilities.

Chapter Two

THE PROBLEM

Researchers have noted that person-centered care leads to improved outcomes for the resident and caregiver (Linzer et al., 2015; Rossi et al., 2015). The general problem is that nurses and CNA thoughts of person-centered care ae unknown (Kusmaul & Waldrop, 2015). This research gap limits knowledge about the individualized care these caregivers are providing. This understanding could contribute to the impact on the delivery of person-centered care in long-term care settings. The residents' view of care received in long-term care facilities is well-researched (Alharbi et al., 2014; Bramley & Matiti, 2014; Ulin et al., 2016). The staff perception of person-centered care and the impact to the nurse and CNA is not well-researched (Donnelly & MacEntee, 2016).

The major segments of this chapter include the literature search strategy, the theoretical foundation, the review of the literature, and a summary of the major themes in the literature. A detail review of literature was necessary to identify the gaps and progress made academically towards the concept of person-centered care. The search was conducted utilizing several library databases and search engines.

Jean Watson's theory of human caring was chosen as the theoretical framework for this study. Person-centered care is directly related to the theory focusing on the human caring experiences (Sitzman & Watson, 2018) and person-centered care is being characterized as a caring feeling (Bramley & Matiti, 2014; Tobiano et al., 2015). A thorough search revealed that the focus had been on the residents' perception of person-centered care (Alharbi et al., 2014a; Bramley & Matiti, 2014; Ulin et al., 2016). This literature review will reveal what was known about person-centered care, the nurses' perception of person-centered care, and the certified nursing assistants' perception of person-centered care. Because these data were limited, a large amount of literature was identified specifically around the general concept of person-centered.

Theoretical Foundation

Watson's caring theory is the theoretical framework that was used for this study (Flagg, 2015). The origin of Watson's theory is centered on how the science of nursing involves a holistic approach which encompasses tuning into one's values and willingness to be committed to caring for others. Watson described caring as a response to a condition of health and wellness. Watson further explained that the nurses' response was characterized by ten carative factors, transpersonal caring relationships and caring moments (Edvardsson et al., 2017). These elements offer caregivers a guide to providing person-centered care. Research on the theory of caring, gives nurses the opportunity to use these factors to enhance communication, which ultimately leads to the effectiveness of professional nursing practice (Brewer & Watson, 2015). The 10 carative factors will be discussed in detail later in the chapter.

The rationale for choosing Jean Watson's theory is directly related to the theory focusing on the human caring experiences (Sitzman & Watson, 2018) and person-centered care is being characterized as a caring feeling (Bramley & Matiti, 2014; Tobiano et al., 2015). Organizations have moved from the practice of providing the nursing staff with scripts when communicating with residents and families (Cleary et al., 2014) to allowing the staff to communicate openly. The caring factor demonstrated by nursing staff has been instrumental in the culture change of an environment based on human caring (Brewer & Watson, 2015). The residents' experienced with human caring revealed that communication and responsiveness to their individual needs left them with a perception that the staff cared more.

These feelings were correlated to trust and dignity (Brewer & Watson, 2015).

Watson's primary writing defines caring as human, attentive and intentional (Watson & Smith, 2002). The caregiver that is intentional is aware of the actions that are implemented. When the nurse is intentional in caring for the resident, a caring relationship between the residents and the nurse is established (Labrague, McEnroe-Petitte, Papathanasiou, Edet, & Arulappan, 2015; Turkel, Watson, & Giovannoni, 2018). The nurse and the resident become comfortable with one another. The caregivers' choices and actions are formulated through the face to face relationship. This caring relationship unifies the nurse and the resident. The connection creates a field of caring patterns .These patterns communicate an authentic caring relationship among the nurse and the residents, (Watson & Smith, 2002).

Person-centered care allows the residents desires and preferences to be brought back into care decisions. Residents have verbalized that it matters to them to have personalized services that are caring (Aiken et al., 2014; Edvardsson, Watt, & Pearce, 2017). The residents wanted to decide when they would awaken and get dress.

They wanted autonomy of what they preferred to like to wear. The choice of incontinence supplies and whether they preferred to be toileted or to wear disposable briefs. The residents were also given options on where and when they would like to dine (Simmons, Durkin, Rahman, Schnelle, & Beuscher, 2014). The residents' experienced with human caring revealed that communication and responsiveness to their individual needs left them with a perception that the staff cared more. These feelings were correlated to trust and dignity (Brewer & Watson, 2015). Services received within a caring environment included the protection of the residents' dignity and stability of their personal autonomy. Caring from the resident's perspective is associated with physical and mental satisfaction (Edvardsson et al., 2017). Utilizing the carative factors of Watson's theory, the fundamental concept of caring has been associated with person-centered care and quality (Edvardsson, 2015).

The Carative Factors and Application to Person-Centered Care

Providing person-centered care is a prominent focus in caring for residents. Consistent with Watson's Theory of Human Caring, person-directed care emphasis the unique strengths, beliefs, and preferences of each resident. Autonomy is promoted while the principles of person-centered care are incorporated (Brown & Bright, 2017). Jean Watson's ten carative factors provide a framework to direct the perception and interpersonal relationship between the resident and the caregiver (Watson, 1985). The primary focus is on the person providing the care as well as the person receiving the care. The carative factors include (Watson, 1979; Turkel et al., 2018).

Watson Theory 10 Carative Factors

Carative Factor 1: Humanistic-Altruistic system of values. The development of a value system that is humanistic and altruistic involves practicing love and kindness (Brown & Bright, 2017). Person-centered care is characterized by the art of caring, which is important to nursing as a profession (Pajnkihar, McKenna, Štiglic, & Vrbnjak, 2017). The caregiver uses eye contact and a gentle touch. Listening is a genuine concern. The resident's primary language is used when communicating. The needs of the resident supersede the task of caring. The caregiver recognizes the resident's potential and limits (Tonin, Nascimento, Lacerda, Favero, Gomes, & Denipote, 2017).

Carative Factor 2: Faith-Hope. The instillation of faith-hope involves providing care based on the residents personal belief systems (Brown & Bright, 2017). Person-centered care emphasizes that the caregiver has a clear understanding of the residents' mind, body and spiritual needs (Pajnkihar et al., 2017). There is harmony with what is desired and what is needed. The caregiver is committed to truly caring. The residents' values are incorporated into daily tasks. There is an opportunity for the resident to reflect on past experiences. The resident is accepted as they are. Dignity and integrity is honored and respected. The residents' previous experiences are recognized and understood (Tonin et al., 2017).

Carative Factor 3: Sensitivity to one's self and to others. The cultivation of sensitivity to one's self and to others involves being aware of your values and beliefs while working on a relationship with others (Brown & Bright, 2017). Person-centered care focuses on caring of an individual as a whole, not just on the caring for the physical resident (Pajnkihar et al., 2017). Self-care is nurtured. The resident is encouraged to exercise their individual desires while the caregiver intentionally prepares to add to the interpersonal relationship. Spiritual practices are allowed and encouraged. The caregiver empowers the resident to practice self-reflection based on their individual preference. This may be accomplished through prayer, meditation, and other forms of expression. If the resident desires to exercise gratitude and forgiveness, through a spiritual ritual, it is allowed. The caregiver remains open and sensitive to the residents' desires (Tonin et al., 2017).

Carative Factor 4: Helping-Trust relationship. The development of a helping, trusting relationship involves being authentic (Brown & Bright, 2017). Person-centered care begins when the caregiver partners with others (Pajnkihar et al., 2017). The partnership with the resident opens opportunity for feelings of caring and compassion to be displayed. Trust becomes a vital part to maintaining the caregiver-resident relationship (Gonzalez, 2017). The caregiver is respectful verbally and nonverbally. The resident is given an opportunity to express their needs at the time they preferred. The caregiver calls the resident by the name the resident requested to be called. Activities provided promote healthy living, freedom, and independence (Tonin et al., 2017).

Carative Factor 5: Positive and negative feelings. The promotion and acceptance of the expression of positive and negative feelings involves affirming the resident's feelings (Brown & Bright, 2017). Person-centered care reduces the desire to treat the resident like an object, leading to residents' dissatisfaction with care (Pajnkihar et al., 2017). The caregiver can reverse this trend by focusing on the residents' psychological, spiritual, and social needs, verses their diagnoses. The caregiver encourages the resident to express their feelings. There is a sense of understanding of what is experienced. Feelings begin to flow among the resident and the caregiver (Tonin et al., 2017).

Carative Factor 6: Creative problem-solving method for decision making. The systematic use of the creative problem-solving method for decision making involves utilizing knowledge to promote healing (Brown and Bright, 2017). Person-centered care is essential to the knowledge, understanding, and acceptance of the caregiver (Pajnkihar et al., 2017). The science of caring to include the methods of application and education directly corresponds with the other. The caregiver assist the resident in identifying meaning to the current situation experienced. Through creativity, the resident express their feelings. The caregiver using intentional touch with permission. The resident becomes aware of their presence with the assistance of the caregiver being authentic (Tonin et al., 2017).

Carative Factor 7: Interpersonal teaching-learning. The promotion of interpersonal teaching and learning involves building a relationship through engagement (Brown & Bright, 2017). Person-centered care empowers self-care. This process is superseded by the perception of competence (Pajnkihar et al., 2017). The caregiver is more aware of the impact health and illness as on the interactions with the resident. This perception is based on education, research, and practice. (Pajnkihar et al., 2017). The resident and caregiver are engaged in teaching and learning exercises. Active listening takes place and acceptance is obtained. The caregiver seeks opportunities to learn from the resident and understand their current world (Tonin et al., 2017).

Carative Factor 8: Healing environment. The provision for a supportive, protective, and/or corrective mental, physical, sociocultural, and spiritual environment involves creating an environment where healing can occur (Brown & Bright, 2017). Person-centered care is provided when the caregiver is able to recognize the internal and external factors that influence the residents' health (Pajnkihar et al., 2017). Needs are supported and the residents' desires are protected. A healing environment is created. Comfort, privacy, and safety are provided. The resident may experience a reconnection between environment and universe. This relinking brings promotes a relationship of respect and integrity (Tonin et al., 2017).

Carative Factor 9: Gratification of human needs. Assistance with the gratification of human needs involves intentionally instituting processes and practices that are person-centered care (Brown & Bright, 2017). Person-centered care emphasizes the importance of recognizing the resident as a human being. Care is provided in a manner that promotes the residents', the spirituality and love for the universe (Pajnkihar et al., 2017). In addition, the caregiver utilizes multiple processes in maintaining the residents' personal awareness. The caregiver respects the needs of the resident and their perception of the world. The residents' needs are anticipated. The art of caring is seen as an honor and privilege (Tonin et al., 2017).

Carative Factor 10: Phenomenological forces. The allowance for existential phenomenological forces involves providing the resident with their person-centered spiritual needs (Brown & Bright, 2017). Person-centered care allows the resident to openly share their beliefs regarding life and death (Pajnkihar et al., 2017). Although the conversation may be sensitive in nature, the caregiver remains present as a listener. The caregiver respects what is important and meaningful to the resident. If the resident prefers a special healing place and time, it is provided. The caregiver respects the residents' beliefs in the unknown, miracles, and the healing power of faith and hope (Tonin et al., 2017).

In Watson's theory, the caregiver and resident is assisted in achieving a harmonious, caring relationship (Watson, 1985). Transactions and behaviors create caring relationships. The theory assumes the act of caring is achieved through the development of an interpersonal relationship between the resident and the caregiver. For this study, the carative factors that will be applicable for the interpretation of the results and the caregivers' perception of person-centered care will be applied during the analysis of the data.

Concept of Person-Centered Care

The concept of person-centered care has been around since the 1980s (Holder, 1983; Holder, 1985; Flagg, 2015; Van Haitsma et al., 2014). Although originally derived from resident and family complaints, the resident was given an opportunity to express specifically what they preferred (Holder, 1983; Tobiano et al., 2015). These preferences and values served as the guide to what was implemented. The long-term care industry has transitioned from institutional care to a more individualized care philosophy. This national movement known as patient-centered care, resident-centered care, or person-centered care, is focused primarily on involving the resident in making decisions regarding their care (Chenoweth et al., 2015; Røen et al., 2017). For purposes of this study we will refer to this change in culture as person-centered care.

Person-centered care has impacted standards of practice in residential facilities (Chenoweth et al., 2015; Røen et al., 2017). This new concept has reduced resident uncertainty through the promotion of culture stability and goal setting (Alharbi et al., 2014). Resulting in a better opportunity to sustain the desired results when implementing this new model. Outcomes of hospital discharges have improved (Ulin et al., 2016). The hospital staff have communicated frequently with the home health agency and nursing home during the patients' hospitalization, rather than at the end of the hospital stay. The person-centered care was provided in partnership with the nursing home. The discharge planning conference occurred within the first 5 days of the hospital stay and included representation from the nursing home. As a result, the residents experienced a lesser number of hospital readmissions. The residents were more capable in coping with their post discharge plan of care (Fålun, Fridlund, Schaufel, Schei, & Norekvål, 2016).

The movement to person-centered care provided residents and staff with the opportunity to become open to alternative forms of care and accommodations (Chenoweth et al., 2015; Røen et al., 2017). The residents were allowed to voice their preferences (Simmons et al., 2014) of when they would like to get out of bed, preference of when to get dress and what they wanted to wear. The residents were also given options regarding incontinence care. These choices were centered on their desired to be toileted or wearing disposable briefs. The residents were also given option on where and when they would like to dine. Alternatives that focused on efficiency, consistency, and decision-making enhanced autonomy and choices. The clinical staff learned to shift their focus from the disease to the resident and the family (Wexler et al., 2015). The medical staff included the residents and family disease management decisions, when there were no other no available interventions. The resident and family became partners in the development of care processes. These interventions influenced staff satisfaction (Chenoweth et al., 2015; Røen et al., 2017).

The desire to have person-centered care has increased, specifically with the elderly population (Song, Scales, Anderson, Wu, & Corazzini, 2018). Research on person-centered care for the resident with dementia has increased over the years (Edvardsson, Sandman, & Borell, 2014). Although the residents had experienced cognitive impairments (Roberts, Morley, Walters, Malta, & Doyle, 2015), they were able to verbalize that when person-centered care was provided, they felt like the staff was more hospitable. It was also noted that the staff appeared to be less stressed, due to knowing what the residents' preferred. When following-up on the residents' needs, the staff reported increased satisfaction, due to being able to provide care they wanted to provide.

Approaches to person-centered care can vary depending on the clinical situation (Elwyn e al., 2014). Motivational interviewing techniques was one method used to accomplish person-centered care. This process encouraged shared decision making, where the resident and the nursing staff made decisions together. The residents reported feeling well informed. The clinician verbalized feelings of organization and prioritization. The residents' family members often served as the experts (Law, Patterson, & Muers, 2017) in expressing the residents' needs, specifically when the resident is unable to express their own desires and preferences. These individuals are accustomed to the residents' daily routines and habits (Barbosa, Sousa, Nolan, & Figueiredo, 2015). The promotion of personhood is directed by the family. The plan of care implemented by the nursing staff are individualized and explicit to the desires of the resident, as informed by the family. The family served as a link between the residents' likings and the care being provided (Tolhurst, & Weicht, 2017).

Person-centered care in long-term care facilities are accommodating more culturally diverse populations (Tayab & Narushima, 2014). Customization of the residents' preferences included understanding the residents' lifestyle and beliefs. This level of understanding recognized that the personal care worker needed to be sensitive to the residents' unique needs, without stereotyping. As a result the caregivers remained culturally competent and the residents received individualized care.

Effect of person-centered care on quality of care. Person-centered care over the last decade has directly been correlated with quality of care (Martínez, Suárez-Álvarez & Yanguas, 2016; Sullivan et al., 2018). This concept in which the caregiver values the resident by treating them as individuals, has been known to be essential to quality care as well as positive outcomes for residents (Flagg, 2015). Person-centered care allows for the residents' perspective to be obtained which includes providing a positive social environment. An environment that was acceptable to the resident's individual needs and desires (Song et al., 2018). For example, nursing staff self-reported that they provided the quality care and activities that the resident preferred after receiving information on how to care for resident with dementia (Edvardsson et al., 2014). Another study reported that nurses felt burnout and depressed while caring for resident with dementia. These feelings impacted the quality of care they provided. However, when developing a person-centered care routine with the residents' families, the nurses felt like they were had provided quality of care to the nursing home residents (Barbosa et al., 2015). Nursing home staff were asked to rate the Advancing Excellence toolkit. The toolkit allowed organizations to enter monthly data, view and compare their progress towards providing person-centered care to nursing home residents. The nursing assistants interviewed the residents about their preferences. The information was then entered into a preprogramed Excel workbook. The interviews by the research assistants revealed that the residents felt that the staff had not met all of their preferences, which led them to believe the care received could have been better. As a result, one hundred percent of the staff revealed that the toolkit provided opportunities to provide quality of care improvements (Van Haitsma et al., 2014).

Research findings have proven the association between registered nurse staffing and improved quality of care (Dellefield, Castle, McGilton, & Spilsbury, 2015). Although the acuity level of the nursing home residents have increased, current federal staffing requirements for Registered Nurses are limited to one RN on duty for at least 8 hours per day, 7 days a week. Studies have reported that increasing the RN staffing to one RN per shift is related to better nursing home quality (Backhaus, Verbeek, van Rossum, Capezuti, & Hamers, 2014; Boyd et al., 2014). A review was conducted of the RN infrastructure (RNs employed in various roles in the nursing home, perceptions of teamwork and open communication) and NH quality (prevalence of pressure ulcers, urinary tract infections, falls, and deficiency citations). Higher RN staffing was associated with a work environment fostering person-centered care as well as improved resident outcomes as evidence by decrease pressure ulcer development, limited restraint use, and decrease readmissions, hence decreasing the organization's operating expenses (Dellefield et al., 2015).

CNAs provide the majority of direct care to the nursing home residents (Kusmaul & Waldrop, 2015). The care they have provided has become important to the receipt of quality care. CNAs that were trained on the concept of person-centered care, provided the **residents** with more choices (Simmons et al., 2014). The principles of person-centered care that uphold the **residents** choices, dignity, self-determination and respect, provides the resident with a purposeful driven life. The researchers suggest a gap regarding how this culture has impacted the daily work of the CNA (Kusmaul & Waldrop, 2015; Tayab & Narushima, 2014).

Effect of person-centered care on quality of life. Person-centered care is a significant factor to quality care (Rodríguez-Martín et al., 2015; Williams, Hadjistavropoulos, Ghandehari, Yao & Lix, 2015). Long-term care facilities have strived to provide excellent quality of care, but frequently the quality of life goes unnoticed (Andrew & Ritchie, 2017). Quality of life can be defined as the perception an individual has regarding culture and value systems (Klapwijk, Caljouw, Pieper, van der Steen, & Achterberg, 2016). The relationship between quality of care and quality of life defines the personal life goals of the resident. The culture shift to person-centered care empowers both the nursing team and the nursing home resident, resulting in improved quality of life (Tayab, & Narushima, 2014).

The enhancement of quality has been contributed by the autonomy given to the residents in making decisions about their lives as well as day to day services being provided to them. Obtaining the resident's perspective is important understanding their quality of life (O'rourke, Fraser, & Duggleby, 2015). Evidence base literature has identified that this concept has not only be measured, but has also been influenced by the behaviors of the individuals caring for the residents (Davila et al., 2016). The residents' quality of life had been impacted by how the staff treated them. There had also been an association between quality of life and the age of the resident, the activities of daily living, pain and disease specific conditions such as dementia psychoses, pulmonary diseases and neurogenic disorders (Klapwijk et al., 2016).

Residents that experienced cognitive deficits, such as dementia, were affected by many quality of life factors (Lloyd et al., 2018). These factors which included irritability, behaviors, and depression escorted the value of person-centered care. These **residents** weren't able to make their own decisions and often times did not have family involvement, therefore the caregivers were expected to be creative in identifying the **residents'** preferences. The knowledge, attitudes, and relationships the caregiver had with the **residents** made the **resident** and family to feel as if the person-centered care methods had been achieved.

Quality of life is subjective and is best defined by the nursing home resident (Seiger, Ternestedt, & Norberg, 2017). Nursing home residents, families and staff from 23 nursing homes across Scotland were asked about their perception of quality of life in a nursing home. The concept of quality of life was different for two of three groups. The family and staff perspectives were similar to each other as they were assessing their QOL if they had been a nursing home resident. Whereas the nursing home resident was reporting their actually feelings. All three groups suggested that caring, supportive staff, and the ability to have some autonomy over food and activities improved their quality of life (Godin, Keefe, Kelloway, & Hirdes, 2015).

In another study, the **residents'** quality of life was directly impacted by the connection they experienced with the staff (Lloyd et al., 2018; O'rourke et al., 2015). The **residents** welcomed the close relationships (Klapwijk et al., 2016). The feelings of togetherness provided a sense of purpose and place. Even when the residents' condition worsened, their quality of life was improved. When compassionate care is provided based on the residents' individualized need, quality is improved (Bramley & Matiti, 2014).

The Person-centered chronic disease management. The concept of self-management and self-care involves the **resident** actively participating in their treatment plan (Dwarswaard, Bakker, van Staa, & Boeije, 2016; Ulin et al., 2016). As with person-centered care, the **resident** has input with medication management, behavioral management, and emotional management. These person-centered care efforts consisted of a collaborative effort between the **resident**, provider, and care givers. The **residents'** input was included in all care activities which resulted in the identification of barriers. Identifying these opportunities early on, offers the **resident** and clinician the opportunity to be more productive. **Residents** reported feelings more satisfied when being offered the opportunity to self-manage their care (Van Haitsma et al., 2014).

Focusing on the **residents'** priorities and preferences is an effective strategy to ensuring person-centered care (Esmaeili, Cheraghi,

& Salsali, 2014). The residents' perception led to an increased awareness of quality of care as well as better residents' satisfaction. Three categories were identified by the p residents as being person-centered: less feelings of uncertainty, care with flexibility, and effective communication. Themes of empathy and decision making were also verbalized. The resident's care plan identified methods for improving person to person interactions and quality of care.

The perception of person-centered care. The act of caring is perceived as essential in the resident experiencing positive outcomes (Desmond et al., 2014). The residents' perception of the caring feelings of the nursing staff has a direct association with the residents' satisfaction and healing (Keeley et al., 2015). These feelings were characterized by the actions of the staff when they were attentive and collaborative with the resident. Additional person-centered care strategies involved listening to the residents carefully as they described their preferences. Residents report that they felt satisfied with the individualized care as a result of the nursing staff providing explanations of the task to be performed, in a manner that the resident understood.

The residents' perception. The most important aspect of

person-centered care is the involvement of the resident (Wexler et al., 2015). The resident viewed person-centered care as receiving nursing care when it was preferred, in a manner that it was preferred (Kehyayan, Hirdes, Tyas, & Stolee, 2015). The resident historically, was not involved in this process. The resident's role was to accept the care that was being delivered, regardless of when it was delivered or how it was delivered. Often times the resident merely sat back and allowed the nursing staff to proceed. Person-centered care places the resident and their preferences in the center of all the services being provided (Donnley & MacIntee, 2016). This theory was characterized by the resident sharing with the nursing staff what mattered most to them. What mattered most varied, depending on the resident's medical condition and decision making ability (Elwyn et al., 2014; (Kehyayan et al., 2015); Been-Dahmen, Dwarswaard, Hazes, Staa, & Ista, 2015).

Kehyayan et al., 2015 identified that the nursing home residents valued a caring environment, preservation of their dignity and having a sense of autonomy. This paradigm shift was necessary in addressing the resident and family concerns as well as assisting the nursing staff in prioritizing the delivery of care (Donnley & MacIntee, 2016). These priorities were very resident specific and consisted of services that the resident saw beneficial and important. The long-term care residents felt like the staff were listening to them. They felt like the staff viewed them as individuals, rather than focusing on their illnesses or disease process (Alharbi et al., 2014). There were reports of less boredom and more autonomy and personal control (Chaudhury, Hung, Rust, & Wu, 2016; Chenoweth et al., 2015; Røen et al., 2017).

The resident is an active participant in management of their day to day treatments to include maintenance and prevention (Been-Dahmen et al., 2015; Kehyayan et al., 2015). The resident prefers person-centered care that is compassionate (Kehyayan et al., 2015). Compassionate care in the eyes of the resident is provided when the care giver knows what they prefer. Services are provided with a caring attitude. The resident desires to be treated as a human being, not a thing (Bramley & Matiti, 2014). The feelings of uncertainty is limited as a result of goal setting that includes the resident's desires (Alharbi et al., 2014).

Residents in long-term care facilities are essentials to the person-centered care process (Esmaeili et al., 2014). These residents have reported that they have received person-centered care (Donnelly & MacEntee, 2016). These feeling are marked by the services received within a caring environment, protection of their dignity, and stability of their personal autonomy. Although the care was personal, the residents reported that they felt distant from the nursing staff because of the nursing staff's workload.

The interest of the resident's perception of person-centered care has increased (Rodríguez-Martín et al., 2015) specifically the impact it has on resident satisfaction. Wilberforce et al., 2016 concluded that there was an association between individualized care and resident satisfaction. Residents who reported feeling they were given decision making control over their care. This positive correlation also demonstrated that residents were more involved in their care when provided with adequate information. Having adequate information regarding care practices made them more satisfied.

The certified nursing assistants' perception. The CNA provides 80% of the direct care in nursing home settings (Gray et al., 2016; Davila et al., 2016). These individuals presume to know more about the residents' desires, than other caregiver (Davila et al., 2016). However, research on the certified nursing assistants' (CNA) perception of person-center care is limited (Halifax, Miaskowski, & Wallhagen, 2018; Kusmaul & Waldrop, 2015; Wilberforce et al.,

2016). As front line staff, attention to nursing assistants' perception need to be highlighted (Halifax et al., 2018). Law & Muers, 2016 suggested that residents received better care when ongoing communication with the caregivers occurred. The resident were clean, comfortable, and happy (Davila et al., 2016). The consistent communication promoted trust among the patient and family members (Barbosa et al., 2015; Law et al., 2017). This partnership promoted attentiveness to the personal needs and desires of family members as well as nursing home residents (Tolhurst, & Weicht, 2017). As a result, the residents received individualized care.

In 2014, Tayab & Narushima revealed a connection of cultural competence and its strong connections to person-centered care. A better trained staff provided an increased opportunity for the CNA to offer the resident culturally-centered choices (Simmons et al., 2014). Although residents may have desired not to be involved directly in their own healthcare discussions, they were very particular about deciding which caregivers would be involved (Bangerter, Van Haitsma, Heid, & Abbott, 2016). The fulfillment of honoring personal care needs were directly associated with the social needs (Andrew & Meeks, 2016).

Although the bulk of the work is being provided by the CNA, the CNAs are seen as being the lowest ranking healthcare professional (Gray et al., 2016). These individuals see themselves as team players that provide quality care. They report being highly satisfied with their jobs. The CNA perceived that the care they provide was special. Research has identified, however, that there was a gap of knowledge between the CNA's perception of person-centered care and the care that was actually being perceived (Hunter, Hadjistavropoulos, & Kaasalainen, 2016; Rodríguez-Martín et al., 2015). Long-term care facilities need to be more engaged to the needs of the nursing assistant (Kusmaul & Waldrop, 2015).

The nurses' perception. The research on the nurse's perception of person-centered care is limited (Wilberforce et al., 2016). Although scarce, research findings suggest that organizational leaders who are knowledgeable of the nurses' perception are more likely to limit barriers that hinder care delivery (Rodríguez-Martín et al., 2015). Being well informed may lead to the development and facilitation of care practices that improve care received by nursing home residents (Rodríguez-Martín et al., 2015).

Family-centered care (FCC), similar to person-centered care, recognizes the family's role in care delivery. According to Foster (2015), the nurse care practices were found to be significantly different from the perception of the family. Findings indicated that the nurses perceived collaborating with families as a barrier to ensuring person-centered care was truly received. Although widely implemented by healthcare organizations, the concept of family-centered care provided nurses with resources necessary in developing family nursing interventions. Nurses recognize that the collaboration with the residents is essential to building a self-management relationship (Kennedy et al., 2014). Old practices have to be discontinued before new practices can be implemented.

The limited research (Van Hooft, Dwarswaard, Jedeloo, Bal & van Staa, 2015) on how nurses perceive person-centered care revealed critical insights and directions aimed at maximizing the effectiveness of the nurses' role in the long-term care setting (Wilberforce et al., 2016). Having insight on these practices could provide leaders with the opportunity to better manage day-to-day operations. Better management may lead to quality improvement initiatives that promote person-centered care practices and job satisfaction (McGilton et al., 2014; Dellefield et al., 2015)

Table 1: *Literature Search (2014 to present)*

Search Engine	Boolean Phrases													Number of Results	Number Used
	nurse perception (person-centered care)	CNA perception (person-centered care)	nurse's perception (other)	CNA's perception (other)	person-centered care	individualized care	patient-centered care	resident-oriented care	nursing homes	residential facilities	green house model	patient focused	carative factors		
CINAHL	0	0	0	0	1	0	0	0	0	0	0	0	0	0	1
Elsevier	0	0	40	0	57	48	698	0	0	24	1	33	0	901	40
Nurs. & Allied Hlth.	0	0	0	0	0	0	0	0	0	0	0	0	0	0	0
ProQuest	0	0	0	0	0	0	1	0	0	0	0	0	1	2	2
PUBMED	0	0	0	0	0	0	0	0	0	0	0	0	1	1	1
SAGE	0	0	19	0	23	14	194	0	0	9	0	8	0	267	20
Science	0	0	0	0	8	5	34	0	87	6	0	8	1	149	10
Wiley	1	0	42	1	27	20	87	0	307	16	5	18	0	524	20
TOTAL	1	0	101	1	115	87	1014	0	394	55	6	67	3	1844	94

Chapter Three

THE DICUSSIONS

Setting

The focus group discussions were held in the conference room of a university located in Virginia. The participants all had experience working in a nursing home that offered a household model of care. The household model offered an intimate living environment that includes features such as private bedrooms, living rooms with fireplaces and private spaces for residents and families to enjoy. The facility featured all private rooms and personal care 24 hours a day, 7 days per week. The person-centered care design promoted family-like relationships as well as independence for the residents. Each resident's schedule was very individualized and based on the residents' preference. There were no personal or organizational conditions that influenced participants, their experience or interpretation of the study results.

Demographics

All of the participants were currently employed at the same nursing home in Chesapeake, Virginia. Focus group 1 consisted of ten female CNA's working 8 hour shifts during the day, evening and night. Focused group 2 consisted of ten LPN's, 1 male and 9 females, working various shifts. Focus group 3 consisted of 5 female RNs working 12 hour shifts during the day and evening or evening and night. All three groups were culturally diverse. The participants' years of experience ranged from one year to greater than 20 years. The participants' ages ranged from early 20s to late 50s. The demographic characteristics of these participants are provided in Table 2.

Table 2: *Characteristics of the Research Participants*

Identifier	Role	Shift	Number of Years working in Long-term Care	Sex	Age band
RN 1	Charge Nurse	Day/Even	5	F	30-39
RN 2	Charge Nurse	Day/Even	15	F	50-59
RN 3	Charge Nurse	Day/Even	12	F	50-59
RN 4	Charge Nurse	Even/Night	20	F	40-49
RN 5	Charge Nurse	Even/Night	25	F	40-49
LPN 1	Primary Nurse	All Shifts	10	F	40-49
LPN 2	Primary Nurse	All Shifts	13	F	40-49
LPN 3	Primary Nurse	All Shifts	2	F	30-39
LPN 4	Primary Nurse	Night	12	F	30-39
LPN 5	Primary Nurse	All Shifts	3	F	40-49
LPN 6	Primary Nurse	All Shifts	9	M	30-39
LPN 7	Primary Nurse	Day/Eve	4	F	30-39
LPN 8	Staff nurse	Day	5	F	30-39
LPN 9	Staff nurse	All Shifts	3	F	30-39
LPN 10	Staff nurse	Evening	3	F	50-59
CNA 1	CNA	All Shifts	2	F	30-39
CNA 2	CNA	All Shifts	5	F	20-29
CNA 3	CNA	Nights	6	F	30-39
CNA 4	CNA	Day	13	F	30-39
CNA 5	CNA	All Shifts	8	F	30-39
CNA 6	CNA	Day	2	F	30-39
CNA 7	CNA	Day/Even	8	F	30-39
CNA 8	CNA	Day	1	F	20-29
CNA 9	CNA	Day	1	F	50-59
CNA 10	CNA	Day	1	F	20-29

Data Collection

The focus group interviews with the 15 nurses and ten CNAs served as the primary means of data collection. To ensure data saturation was obtained, the researcher added an additional focus group, bringing the participants to 25 versus the original plan of having 20 participants. Following the official IRB approval on October 5, 2018 (10-05-18-0350565), the researcher submitted the Invitation to participate to the organizations' Administrator (see Appendix C). The Administrator submitted the document to all nurses and Certified Nursing Assistants and instructed those who were interested in participating to contact the researcher directly. The researcher received 25 correspondences of interests over a two-week period of time.

The focus group discussions were held in a conference room of a local university. The room consisted of a long oval conference table that could accommodate 12 people. The focus groups were held in the same location on three different dates and times. The duration of the semi structured interviews were approximately 60 minutes each session. The potential participants' direct correspondence with the researcher and the off-site interview location denoted that there was not a need for a letter of cooperation from the organization.

The researcher began the discussion with an explanation of the purpose of the study, importance and expectations for all participants. The IRB approved informed consent was distributed and discussed. After signing the consent, each participants' was identity was protected by assigning a code. The participants were given an individual index card identifying their role and a corresponding number. The researcher documented the demographic data utilizing the participant's code (see Table 2). Participants were informed that their personal opinions and views on person-centered care were very important to the study and that there were no right or wrong responses. The researcher also reminded the participants that the conversations would be audio recorded. The focus group were asked the following questions:

1. Tell me about the care residents received here.

2. What is your understanding of person-centered care?

3. How do you know that you have provided person-centered care?

The researcher recorded all group sessions utilizing a voice recorder cellphone application. Prior to responding to each question, the participants announced their participant code which included their respective positions and assigned number. Each recording was saved and labeled as Focus Group 1, 2 or 3. The recordings were then transferred from the cell phone to a password protected USB drive. There were no variations in the anticipated data collection plan. There were no unusual circumstances encountered during data collection.

Data Analysis

Digital recordings of the interviews were listened by the researcher immediately after each focus group session interviews. The recording were then electronically submitted to the Nvivo transcription program. The program transcribed the recorded sessions into a word document arranged based on the corresponding question asked. Interview recordings were transcribed verbatim. The transcript for each session was shared with each individual participate to ensure accuracy. No variations or corrections were needed.

Description of Themes

Microsoft Word paragraph styles were applied to the transcripts. The transcripts were then loaded into the Nvivo12 Plus qualitative data management program. Line by line automatic coding was conducted of the participants' responses. The thematic framework was used to ensure that the generated themes correlated with the original transcripts. The reanalyzing of this data assisted in an accurate interpretation of the findings. The cluster of data, similar phrases, and sentences extracted two overarching themes: resident preferences and caring approaches (see table 3).

Table 3: *Percentage of Theme Content*

Themes	Data Coverage Percentage		
	Care Residents Receive	Understanding of PCC	Knowledge that PCC was Provided
Resident preferences	23%	41%	36%
Caring approaches	38%	53%	9%

Description of Carative Factor Themes

The researcher created three main source files that corresponded with each interview question. Ten subgroups (nodes) were created for each interview question. The subgroups represented Watson's 10 carative factors. Codes and references emerged from the three source folders signifying the interview questions. The codes represented the number of sources and the references represented amount of content derived from the participant responses. The responses to the three interview questions identified a total of seventy-five codes and 356 references (see Table 4). No further interviews were required, as data saturation had occurred.

Table 4: *Codes and References*

Source File	Code	References
Care Residents Receive	25	116
Understanding of PCC	25	94
Knowledge that PCC was Provided	25	146
Total	75	356

For each response, the researcher noted the main ideas that occurred in the responses. The main ideas were then reviewed for reoccurrence. Three main themes were identified from the reoccurring main ideas. The themes materialized from the interview questions included sensitivity to self, creative decision making, and expression of feelings (see Table 5). There were no discrepant cases.

Table 5: *Percentage of Theoretical Theme Content per Interview Question*

Carative Factors	The Care Received	Understanding of PCC	Knowledge of PCC Provided
Love and Kindness	1.03%	0.00%	21.20%
Faith and Hope	0.00%	0.96%	4.16%
Sensitivity to Self	41.07%	28.17%	4.34%
Trusting Relationships	4.70%	17.05%	9.25%
Expression of Feelings	19.27%	6.89%	34.76%
Creative Decision Making	17.57%	40.64%	14.84%
Teaching and Learning	12.09%	4.28%	10.00%
Healing Environment	4.27%	0.96%	1.45%
Gratification	0.00%	1.05%	0.00%
Phenomenological Beliefs	0.00%	0.00%	0.00%

Sensitivity to Self

The first interview question about the care the residents received revealed a main theme of sensitivity to the patients' desires with a content coverage of 41% (see Table 6). The word frequency query revealed two categories referencing general care activities at 86 words and personal centered care at 36 words (see Table 7). Fifty-one percent of sensitivity content was provided by the LPNs, 33% by the

CNAs, and 16% was provided by the RNs (See Table 10). The cultivation of sensitivity to one's self and to others involved the caregiver being aware of the residents' value and beliefs and caring for the resident as a whole (Brown & Bright, 2017; Pajnkihar et al., 2017).

RN3: We go by the resident's desires.

LPN4: I focused on making sure the residents received their medication at the time they prefer it. Its more resident centered when there's a lower number of residents to provide care for.

CNA5: I bathe them and make their food. I cooked the food for them the way they prefer it.

Table 6: *The Care Residents Received Word Query*

Word	Count	Similar Words
activities	86	activities, assistance, bathing, breath, building, care, charge, coaching, conduct, dining, doctor, dressing, eating, education, feeding, feel, going, house, keeping, last, live, look, love, model, nursing, passing, post, review, seeking, service, share, short, sleeping, start, training, try, use, walk, work, worst
personal	36	advocate, better, card, day, diabetic, doctor, family, independent, intellectual, model, nurse, personal, post, self, service, someone, star, tell, transfer, worker

Creative problem solving for decision making

The second interview question about the caregivers understanding of PCC revealed a main theme of creative decision making methods with a content coverage of 41 percent (see Table 5). The word frequency query revealed two categories referencing wanted care at 49 words and individualized care at 24 words. Sixty-four percent of creative decision making content was provided by the LPNs, nineteen percent provided by the RNs, and seventeen percent by the CNAs (See Table 9). The resident acknowledges and accepts the care provided as authentic and meaningful (Tonin et al., 2017).

RN1: The care is targeted at meeting the needs of the resident.

LPN3: Repeating tasks even if you know that you already provided them, just to please the resident.

CNA7: Treat the resident as an individual.

Table 7: *The Understanding of PCC Word Query*

Word	Count	Similar Words
Individualized care	24	advocate, chief, contractor, day, family, individual, individualized, individuals, life, pain, person, personal, someone
Wanted care	49	care, desires, loved, needs, please, want, wants, wishes

Expression of feelings

The third interview question about the caregivers understanding of PCC revealed a main theme specific to expression of feelings with a content coverage of 35 percent (see Table 6). The word frequency query revealed two categories referencing affection at 50 words and preferences at 17 words (See Table 9). Forty-six percent of expression of feelings content was provided by the CNAs, twenty-seven percent by the LPNs, and twenty-seven percent was provided by the RNs (See Table 10). The promotion and acceptance of the expression of positive and negative feelings involves the caregiver acknowledging the resident's feelings (Brown & Bright, 2017). Feelings begin to flow among the resident and the caregivers (Tonin et al., 2017).

> RN1: The resident completed the satisfaction surveys with all positive comments. The resident request that I am the caregiver.

LPN3: Lots of residents fuss with the nurses and try to tell them how they are feeling. I listen. I give a listening ear.

CNA10: The resident lights up when they see you.

Table 8: *Knowledge that PCC had been Provided Word Query*

Word	Count	Similar Words
Affection	50	caregiver, family, great job, light, love, person, personally, playing, tell, alert, feeling, feelings, job, light, lot, love, need, note, recognition, cry, listening, thank you, glad, satisfaction surveys, caregiver, families, family, house, person, present, song, care positive, comments request extra mile verbalize aren't complaining call lights acknowledges pleased good goodies relaxing
Preference	17	determine needs, assessment, findings, plan, specific, desires, centered care, step back, asking, prefers, tells, call, want, goals

Table 9: *Percentage of Theme Content per Participant Category*

	Percent of Content		
Participant Category	Sensitivity to Desires	Creative Decision Making	Expression of Feelings
RN	16%	19%	27%
LPN	51%	64%	27%
CNA	33%	17%	46%

Evidence of Trustworthiness

The credibility of the study was established through triangulation and saturation. Triangulation was obtained when the focus group participants openly shared their personal stories and experiences, increasing more validity (Carter et al., 2014; Fusch & Ness, 2015). Data saturation was obtained with the focus groups participants providing a variety of perspectives based on their individual exposure. Focus group 1 consisted of 10 CNA's, group 2 consisted of ten LPN's, and group 3 consisted of 5 RNs. All groups were within the recommended focus group size of 5-12 (Cheng, 2014; Kai-wen, 2014; Fusch & Ness, 2015). The researcher's experience as a Nurse and CNA offered open relationship with the participants. The participants provided detailed, in depth information on person-centered care resulting in a broader understanding of the person-centered care phenomenon (Rauf et al., 2014; Carter et al., 2014). The researcher utilized the responses obtained from the face to face focus group sessions and the audio-tape. The validity was strengthened with each participant cross validating their individual transcripts. Thematic analysis, multiple coding, was implemented to preserve the validity of the data.

The transferability of the study was obtained through minimizing the generalization of ethical thoughts and judgement with a variation in the selection of the study participants (Leviton, 2017; Wilson, 2016). I collected data from a diverse range of nurses and CNAs with long-term care experience of a minimum of one year. The participants varied in color, race, ethnicity, and national origin.

The dependability of the study was established through audit trails and triangulation. The use of this method provided for reliability through consistency (Darawsheh, 2014; Leung, 2015). The researcher compared the audio taped data to the Nvivo transcriptions. To add to the reliability of the data, the researcher asked each group the same questions in the same order.

The confirmability was established through reflexivity (Darawsheh, 2014; Hoover & Morrow, 2015). The researcher as the instrument for the study recognized that her experiences as a Registered Nurse and CNA were motivators to the implementation of the research study.

Chapter Four

THE PERCEPTION

The researcher asked three exploration questions that served as the core interview questions for the focus group sessions (Cheng, 2014). As presented in Table 6, the first exploration question supported the Research Question 1. The second exploration questions supported Research Question 2. The following research questions were explored using a focus group design.

Research Question 1-

What is the nurses' and CNA's perception of person-centered care?

Research Question 2-

What are the carative factors that influence the nurse and CNA's perception of person-centered care?

Table 10: *Research Questions and Interview Questions*

Research Questions		Interview Questions
RQ1	What is the nurses' and CNA's perception of person-centered care?	1. Tell me about the care residents received here.
RQ2	What are the carative factors that influence the nurse and CNA's perception of person-centered care?	2. What is your understanding of person-centered care? 3. How do you know that you have provided person-centered care?

Themes

Theme 1: Resident preferences. The participants expressed the importance of providing care as preferred by the resident and families (see Table 11). The residents' plan of care, to include their goals, were to be recognized and honored. The significance of listening to the resident as well as their designated representative was vital to meeting the individualized needs. Participants also identified that involving the resident in care decisions supported their attempt to provide person-centered care. Caregivers do not know what the resident prefers unless they are informed directly by the family or the resident. Asking about preferences was the primary means of identifying what was desired.

Table 11: *The nurse perception of person-centered care*

Theme	Data clusters	Sample statements from participants
Resident Preferences	wants	
	care preferred	The resident request that I am the caregiver because I provide care they prefer.
	resident goals	
	preference	Sometimes you don't know if you are providing resident-centered care, unless you ask the resident.
	self-care needs	
	needs identified	The resident goals are met.
	ask	The resident light up when they see you because they prefer you.
	desire	I provided treatments for post-op residents the way they want it.
	individualized	
	plan	Direct resident care, splinting, resident education about self-care, as they desire it.
		Try to keep the residents independence, they want to be.
		When the resident request things you try to provide it.
		The care and treatment plan is based on the wants and needs of the individual.

Theme 2: Caring approach. The participants verbalized that using a caring approach when delivering care was a main factor in their perception of person-centered care (see Table 12). The residents would often show gratitude when the caregiver's took time to listen and talk with them. Participants reported that the residents' expression of gratitude made caregiver feel like the care was sufficient as well as person-centered. The residents wanted care that was empathetic, nice, and compassionate. When care was provided in this manner, the resident and families were happy. The satisfied residents were pleased to see the caregivers and would often request to receive care by them. These requests resulted in the caregivers' perception that person-centered care must have been provided, since the resident and family were pleased. The participants voiced that exhibiting a friendly, caring approach was seen as providing person-centered care.

Table 12: *A description of theme two: A Caring Approach.*

Caring approach	listen	I listen.
	assist	I give a listening ear
	closeness	Assist with feeding resident, bathing and transferring the resident; I take my time.
	talk	
	pain	Person-centered care gives you a closeness with the resident
	touch	
	soft spoken	I talk with the resident while I am passing medications and providing wound care treatments
	patience	I am patient when I provide treatments, administered medication, trach care, and wound care.
	empathy	

The nurses' and CNA's perception of person-centered care. The focus groups were asked the first interview question about the care the residents received while living in the nursing home. The common theme identified was that the residents received care that was a combination of what the caregivers were required to routinely provide and care specific to what the residents requested. Sixty-seven percent of the nurses reported that the residents received assessments, medications, and treatments. Fourteen percent (3 nurses) reported that the resident receive specific tasks as they request them or as their family request them. Twenty percent (2 nurses) reported that they provide a combination of routine task and task specific to the residents' request (see Figure 2). Ninety percent (9 CNAs) reported that the resident received assistance with bathing, dressing, feedings, and transfers (ADLs). Ten percent (1 CNA) reported serving as a resident advocate to ensure the resident needs were met (see Table 13).

Table 13: *The nurse description of person-centered care.*

Participants	Statement	Providing Routine Care with compassion	Resident and/or Family Requested Care
RN1	"I assess the residents' ability to perform routine activities of daily living to include bathing, dressing and eating."	X	
RN2	I resident and family receive specific education to keep them out of the emergency room	X	X
RN3	"We go by the residents desires"		X
RN4	"I pass medications and providing wound care treatments. I assess the resident."	X	
RN5	"Serve as the charge nurse. I ensure the CNA's are providing person-centered care based on the residents' needs."	X	X
LPN1	Provided treatments and care for residents needed medications.	X	
LPN2	Assist residents to the dining and TV area.	X	

LPN3	I focused on making sure the residents received their medication on time.	X		
LPN4	I provide care centered around the care the family wanted		X	
LPN5	I provided treatments	X		
LPN6	I care for residents have been on their last breath, hospice, and those who need wound care	X		
LPN7	I provide vent, trach, and wound care. I provide diabetic rounds, skilled care.	X		
LPN8	I handle emergencies and pass medications	X		
LPN9	We have to remember the residents are still people.		X	
LPN10	Medication reviews, trach care, talking to the doctor	X		

Table 14: *The CNA's description of person-centered care.*

Participants	Statement	Routine CNA Care with Compassion	Resident/Family Requested Care
CNA1	"We prepare them for bed."	X	
CNA2	"The resident receives ADLs and comfort"	X	
CNA3	"They receive direct resident care, splinting and education about self-care."	X	
CNA4	"I assist with catheter and wound care."	X	
CNA5	"I serve as a resident advocate in making sure their needs are addressed."		X
CNA6	"I assist in feeding, bathing and transferring the residents."	X	
CNA7	"They receive assistance with their ADLs."	X	
CNA8	"I assist with ADLS and transferring them."	X	
CNA9	"I bath them, make their food. We cooked the food for them as well."	X	
CNA10	"I assist the resident when they start to wander off the unit."	X	

The carative factors that influence the perception of person-centered care. The focus groups were asked the second interview question about their understanding of PCC. The discussions revealed that eight carative factors influenced their understanding, with the main factor being the creative problem-solving method for decision making at 41 percent (see table 4). The nurses reported that their understanding of PCC was influenced by seven carative factors with the main factor as creative decision making. The CNAs reported that their understanding of PCC was influenced by five carative factors with the main factor being sensitivity to self (see Table11).

Table 15: *Understanding of PCC*

Carative Factors	CNAs	RN	LPN
Love and Kindness	0.00%	0.00%	00.00%
Faith and Hope	4.00%	12.50%	0.00%
Sensitivity to Self	37.00%	10.75%	15.00%
Trusting Relationships	32.00%	15%	3.50%
Expression of Feelings	10.00%	13%	10.00%
Creative Decision Making	17.00%	19.00%	64.00%
Teaching and Learning	0.00%	13.75	2.25%
Healing Environment	0.00%	16.00	2.75&
Gratification	0.00%	0.00%	2.50%
Phenomenological Beliefs	0.00%	0.00%	0.00%

The focus groups were asked the third interview question about how did they know PCC had been provided. The discussions revealed the influence of eight carative factors, with the main factor being the expression of feelings at 35 percent (see Table 4). The LPNs reported that they knew PCC was being provided through Teaching and Learning. The RNs and CNAs reported that they knew PCC had been provided when the expression of feelings were shared (see Table 11).

Table 16: *Knowledge of PCC Provided*

Carative Factors	CNAs	RN	LPN
Love and Kindness	30.00%	23.25%	5.00%
Faith and Hope	1.00%	22.25%	1.00%
Sensitivity to Self	5.25%	0.00%	0.00%
Trusting Relationships	15.00%	0.00%	3.00%
Expression of Feelings	46.00%	27.00%	27.00%
Creative Decision Making	0.00%	27.50%	28.75%
Teaching and Learning	0.00%	0.00%	35.00%
Healing Environment	2.75%	0.00%	0.25%
Gratification	0.00%	0.00%	0.00%
Phenomenological Beliefs	0.00%	0.00%	0.00%

Summary

Twenty-five participants were included in the study, 5 RNs, 10 LPNs, and 10 CNAs. As seen in Table 2, most of the participants were females, all of whom had worked a minimum of one year in a long-term care setting. The CNA participants had worked an average of 4.7 years and the nurses (RNs and LPNs) worked an average of 9.4 years. The participants' ages ranged from early 20s to late 50s. The analysis of the three interview questions uncovered three main themes factors including sensitivity to self, creative decision making, and expression of feelings. The response to RQ1 revealed that 67 percent of the nurses and ninety percent of the CNAs described their perception of person-centered care as showing providing routine care in a caring and compassionate manner. The response to RQ2 revealed that eight carative factors influenced the nurses and CNAs perception of person-centered care. In chapter 5 I will interrupt the study findings, describe the limitations of the study and recommendation for further research. The chapter will close with the limitations and conclusion.

Chapter Five

THE INTERPRETATION

In this study, the nurse's and CNA's perception of the person-centered care was explored. The nature of the study addressed the research gap through a qualitative approach with focused group discussions. The study was conducted to discover the nurses' and CNAs' perception of person-centered care and the carative factors that influence their perception. When the nursing home residents' unique needs are understood, the residents' quality of life is improved (Desmond et al., 2014; Linzer et al., 2015; Rodríguez-Martín et al., 2015; Rossi et al., 2015). The findings revealed that the nurses' and CNA's perception of person-centered care was viewed as providing services with a caring and compassionate manner. The study also identified that eight carative factors influenced the nurses and CNAs perception of person-centered care.

Interpretation of Findings

The nurses and CNA's of this study agreed with the finding identified by Wexler et al., 2015, that the most important aspect of person-centered care is the involvement of the resident. Kehyayan et al., 2015 along with the participants in this study, recognized that the nursing home residents valued a caring environment and they wanted to be listened to carefully. The purpose of this study was to explore the nurses and CNAs perception of person-centered care and to identify the carative factors that influence person-centered care. The study revealed that the Nurses and CNAs perception of person-centered care was specific to how the care was being delivered. Eight of the ten carative factors were identified as influential in their perception of person-centered care. These factors included Carative Factor 2: Faith-hope, Carative Factor 3: Sensitivity to one's self and to others, Carative Factor 4: Helping-trust relationship, Carative Factor 5: Positive and negative feelings, Carative Factor 6: Creative Problem-solving method for decision making, Carative Factor 7: Interpersonal teaching-learning, Carative Factor 8: Healing Environment, Carative Factor 9: Gratification of human needs, and forces. The factors that were excluded were Carative Factor #1- Humanistic-altruistic system of values and Carative Factor 10: Phenomenological

The nurses' and CNA's perception of person-centered care

Donnelly and MacEntee (2016) revealed that residents have reported receiving person-centered care when the caregiver provided a caring environment and protected their dignity. The nurses and CNAs of this study supported this finding when they verbalized that their perception of received person-centered care was assisting the resident with bathing, dressing, and activities of daily living in a caring and comforting manner. The nurses reported that the residents received person-centered care while medications and treatments were being administered because they took their time to ensure that care was being provided as ordered by the physician. The CNAs stated that when person-centered care was provided, the residents would be glad to see them the next day, the families would write a personal thank you note or share with the manager how pleased they were with the care. The nurses and CNAs of the study acknowledged, as stated in previous research, that relationships were built with the residents while daily care was being provided (McGilton et al., 2014). The person-centered care environment encouraged the residents to openly communicate their desires and wishes. As supported by Simmons et al., 2014, the residents' family members also shared the preferences and values of their loved ones with the staff as well. The CNAs validated, as reported by other researchers, that the residents were given alternative forms of care and accommodations (Chenoweth et al., 2015; Røen et al., 2017), such as receiving their bath and having their meals prepared by the

CNA. The residents verbalized what they would have for breakfast and where they would eat the meal, promoting a sense of autonomy as revealed by Brewer & Watson (2015). Unlike the findings conveyed by Esmaeili, Cheraghi, and Salsali (2014), the perception of person-centered care as reported by the participants was not specific to the preferences or the desires of the resident. The nurses and CNAs of this study validated by verbalizing that they knew person-centered care was provided when the residents and families expressed gratification for the services. The care was not specific to a requests, but was provided with compassion and a caring attitude. As a result of the caring attitude, the residents and families expressed gratitude. These expressions were translated into nurses and CNAs perception that person-centered care had been provided.

The carative factors that influence the perception of person-centered care

The study conducted by Brown and Bright (2017) revealed that care provided on *faith-hope* was based on the resident's personal belief systems. The participants of this study shared that the residents openly shared their personal thoughts and beliefs. The CNAs reported that the residents were encouraged to be as independent as possible, as researched by (Tonin et al., 2017), *self-care* was encouraged. The residents would assist in choosing the times they would prefer their baths. The nurses and CNAs believed, just as Gonzalez (2017), that a *trust* was a vital part to maintaining the caregiver-resident relationship. The nurses discussed that the residents and families trusted that the care was being provided per the physicians' orders. The residents were encouraged to *express their feelings*. The CNAs conveyed that the residents were least likely to complain when they felt the caregiver was not rushing to provide care, as recounted by Tonin et al., 2017. The nurses reported that *education* was provided to the patient and their family members. Information on medication and treatments was provided during the care plan meetings. These interactions assisted in building relationships (Brown & Bright, 2017). According to Pajnkihar et al., 2017, the caregiver should be open to the *internal and external factors* that influence the residents' health. The nurses and CNAs shared that they would often take the time to play games and listen to music with the residents. These moments spent with the resident created a healing environment as residents appeared to be more relaxed when care was being provided. Person-centered care meant that the resident was a human being with real *human needs*, feelings and emotions (Tonin et al., 2017). The nurses and the CNAs verbalized that they attempted to respect the residents' *personal awareness*, as revealed also by Tonin et al., 2017. At times, the resident would share stories about how things used to be when they were younger.

The primary carative factor that influence the perception of person-centered care was the nurses and CNAs use of *knowledge to promote healing*. The residents reported that they felt satisfied with the individualized care as a result of the nursing staff providing explanations of the task to be performed, in a manner that the resident understood. As reported by Keeley et al., 2015, the participants verbalized that the residents' perception of the caring feelings of the nursing staff were directly associated with the residents' satisfaction. The nurses shared that the residents who were satisfied were healthier than the residents who complained more about their care. The residents who were pleased with the care they received were more pleasant when communicating with the staff, as confirmed by Davila et al., 2016. The nurses and CNAs supported the findings of Desmond et al., 2014, by verbalizing that the act of caring that was perceived by the residents caused positive outcomes. These feelings were characterized by the actions of the staff when they were attentive and collaborative with the resident, as studied by Keeley et al., 2015.

Chapter Six

THE IMPACT

The findings from this study have the potential to impact positive social change at the organizational level, influencing the delivery of care within long-term care settings. The study addressed the research gap of the nurses' and CNA's thoughts of the person-centered care services they deliver. The findings provided a better understanding of how person-centered care was perceived by the caregiver. The nurses and CNAs perception of person-centered care was specific to providing services in a caring and compassionate manner. The care provided was not specific to the residents' preference or request, but was perceived as person-centered based on how the care had been delivered.

The theoretical implications of Jean Watson's theory of caring may contribute to the knowledge of nursing practice. The nurses and CNAs reported that the use of knowledge while communicating with the resident was a significant factor that influenced their perception of person-centered care. When they were attentive and collaborative, the residents were happier, more satisfied (Keeley et al., 2015). The satisfied residents complained less and were healthier.

Long-term care facilities should include the delivery of person-centered care as a major component of new employee orientation and their annual education program for nurses and CNAs. This study highlights the importance of providing long-term care residents with services that are caring and compassionate. The study also provided an understanding that nurse and CNAs perceived that creatively including the resident in decision making was a major factor in providing person-centered care. Ongoing research to substantiate the effectiveness of the nurses and CNAs perception of person-centered care in long-term care would be beneficial.

Conclusion

Person-centered care includes the caring and compassionate approach taken when care is being delivered. The nurse and CNA participants in the study highlighted the importance of including the resident in decision making through communicating openly and developing relationships. Implementation of these strategies appeared to be satisfying to the resident. On the other hand, nurses and CNAs also need time and resources to establish such caring environments.

REFERENCES

Abbott, K. M., Heid, A. R., & Van Haitsma, K. (2016). We can't provide season tickets to the opera: Staff perceptions of providing preference-based, person-centered care. *Clinical Gerontologist,* 39(3), 190-209.

Aiken L., Rafferty A. & Sermeus W. (2014) Caring nurses hit by a quality storm. *Nursing Standard, 28, 22–25.*

Alharbi, T. S. J., Olsson, L. E., Ekman, I., & Carlström, E. (2014). The impact of organizational culture on the outcome of hospital care: After the implementation of person-centered care. *Scandinavian Journal of Public Health,* 42(1), 104-110

Alharbi, T. S. J., Carlström, E., Ekman, I., Jarneborn, A., & Olsson, L. E. (2014a). Experiences of person-centered care-patients' perceptions: Qualitative study. *BMC Nursing,* 13(1), 1.

Andrew, A., & Ritchie, L. (2017). Culture change in aged-care facilities: A café's contribution to transforming the physical and social environment. *Journal of Housing for the Elderly*, 31(1), 34-46.

Andrew, N., & Meeks, S. (2016). Fulfilled preferences, perceived control, life satisfaction, and loneliness in elderly long-term care residents. *Aging & Mental Health,* 1-7.

Bachnick, S., Ausserhofer, D., Baernholdt, M., Simon, M., & Match RN study group. (2018). Patient-centered care, nurse work environment and implicit rationing of nursing care in Swiss acute care hospitals: A cross-sectional multi-center study. *International Journal of Nursing Studies*, 81, 98-106.

Backhaus, R., Verbeek, H., van Rossum, E., Capezuti, E., & Hamers, J.P.H. (2014). Nurse staffing impact on quality of care in nursing homes: A systematic review of longitudinal studies. *Journal of the American Medical Directors Association*, 15(6), 383-393.

Bangerter, L. R., Van Haitsma, K., Heid, A. R., & Abbott, K. (2016). Make me feel at ease and at home: Differential care preferences of nursing home residents. *The Gerontologist,* 56(4), 702-713.

Baumeister, R. F., Ainsworth, S. E., & Vohs, K. D. (2016). Are groups more or less than the sum of their members: The moderating role of individual identification. *Behavioral and Brain Sciences,* 39.

Barbosa, A., Sousa, L., Nolan, M., & Figueiredo, D. (2015). Effects of person-centered care approaches to dementia care on staff: a systematic review. *American Journal of Alzheimer's Disease & Other Dementias,* 30(8), 713-722.

Been-Dahmen, J. M., Dwarswaard, J., Hazes, J. M., Staa, A., & Ista, E. (2015). Nurses' views on patient self-management: a qualitative study. *Journal of Advanced Nursing,* 71(12), *2834-2845.*

Bell, E., Campbell, S., & Goldberg, L. R. (2015). Nursing identity and patient- centeredness in scholarly health services research: a computational text analysis of PubMed abstracts 1986–2013. *BMC health services research,* 15(1), 3.

Boyd, M., Armstrong, D., Parker, J., Pilcher, C., Zhou, L., McKenzie-Green, B., & Connolly, M.J. (2014). Do gerontology nurse specialists make a difference in hospitalization of long-term care residents: Results of a randomized comparison trial. *Journal of the American Geriatrics Society,* 62(10), 1962-1967.

Bramley, D. (2015). Using focus groups for ELT research. *Osaka Journal of Advance Language Teaching, 98.*

Bramley, L., & Matiti, M. (2014). How does it really feel to be in my shoes: Patients' experiences of compassion within nursing care and their perceptions of developing compassionate nurses. *Journal of Clinical Nursing,* 23(19-20), 2790-2799.

Brewer, B. B., & Watson, J. (2015). Evaluation of authentic human caring professional practices. *Journal of Nursing Administration,* 45(12), 622- 627.

Broomfield, R. (2014). A nurse's guide to qualitative research. *Australian Journal of Advanced Nursing,* 32(3).

Carter, N., Bryant-Lukosius, D., DiCenso, A., Blythe, J., & Neville, A. J. (2014). The use of triangulation in qualitative research. *Oncology Nursing Forum,* 41(5).

Chaudhury, H., Hung, L., Rust, T., & Wu, S. (2016). Do physical environmental changes make a difference: Supporting person-centered care at mealtimes in nursing homes. *Dementia,* 16(7), 878-896.

Chatchumni, M., Namvongprom, A., Sandborgh, M., Mazaheri, M., & Eriksson, H. (2015). Nurses' perceptions of patients in pain and pain management: a focus group study in Thailand. *Pacific Rim international Journal of Nursing Research,* 19(2), 164-177.

Cheng, K. W. (2014). A study on applying focus group interview on education. *Reading Improvement,* 51(4), 381-385.

Chenoweth, L., Jeon, Y. H., Stein-Parbury, J., Forbes, I., Fleming, R., Cook, J., & Tinslay, L. (2015). PerCEN trial participant perspectives on the implementation and outcomes of person-centered dementia care and environments. *International Psychogeriatrics,* 27(12), 2045-2057.

Ciemins, E. L., Brant, J., Kersten, D., Mullette, E., & Dickerson, D. (2015). A qualitative analysis of patient and family perspectives of palliative care. *Journal of Palliative Medicine, 18(3),* 282-285.

Cleary, M., Horsfall, J., & Hayter, M. (2014). Data collection and sampling in qualitative research: does size matter. *Journal of Advanced Nursing,* 70(3), 473-475.

Creswell, J. W., & Creswell, J. D. (2017). Research design: Qualitative, quantitative, and mixed methods approaches. Sage publications.

Davila, H., Abrahamson, K., Mueller, C., Inui, T. S., Black, A. G., & Arling, G. (2016). Nursing assistant perceptions of their role in quality improvement processes in nursing homes. *Journal of*

Nursing Care Quality, 31(3), 282-289.

Darawsheh, W. (2014). Reflexivity in research: Promoting rigor, reliability and validity in qualitative research. *International Journal of Therapy and Rehabilitation,* 21(12), 560-568.

Dellefield, M. E., Castle, N. G., McGilton, K. S., & Spilsbury, K. (2015). The relationship between registered nurses and nursing home quality: An integrative review (2008-2014). *Nursing Economics, 33(2), 95.*

Desmond, M. E., Horn, S., Keith, K., Kelby, S., Ryan, L., & Smith, J. (2014). Incorporating caring theory into personal and professional nursing practice to improve perception of care. *International Journal for Human Caring, 18(1),* 35-44.

Donnelly, L., & MacEntee, M. I. (2016). Care perceptions among residents of LTC facilities purporting to offer person-centered care. *Canadian Journal on Aging/La Revue canadienne du vieillissement, 35(2), 149-160.*

Drake, J. (2016). *Tools that measure caring: A systematic literature review of the impact of caring* (Doctoral dissertation). Retrieved from Walden Dissertations and Doctoral Studies Collection at Scholar Works.

Duprez, V., Vandecasteele, T., Verhaeghe, S., Beeckman, D., & Van Hecke, A. (2017). The effectiveness of interventions to enhance self-management support competencies in the nursing profession: a systematic review. *Journal of advanced nursing,* 73(8), 1807-1824.

Dwarswaard, J., Bakker, E. J., van Staa, A., & Boeije, H. R. (2016). Self-management support from the perspective of patients with a chronic condition: a thematic synthesis of qualitative studies. *Health Expectations,* 19(2), 194-208.

Edvardsson, D., Sandman, P. O., & Borell, L. (2014). Implementing national guidelines for person centered care of people with dementia in residential aged care: Effects on perceived person-centeredness, staff strain, and stress ofconscience. *International Psychogeriatrics,* 26(7), 1171-9.

Edvardsson D. (2015) Notes on person-centered care: what it is and what it is not. Nordic *Journal of Nursing Research,* 35, 65–66.

Edvardsson, D., Watt, E., & Pearce, F. (2017). Patient experiences of caring and person centeredness are associated with perceived nursing care quality. *Journal of Advanced Nursing,* 73(1), 217-227.

Elwyn, G., Dehlendorf, C., Epstein, R. M., Marrin, K., White, J., & Frosch, D. L. (2014). Shared decision making and motivational interviewing: Achieving patient-centered care across the spectrum of health care problems. *The Annals of Family Medicine,* 12(3), 270-275.

Esmaeili M, Cheraghi MA, Salsali M. (2014) Cardiac patients' perception of patient centered care: A qualitative study. *Nursing in Critical Care,* 21(2), 97-104.

Ervin, A. M., Taylor, H. A., & Ehrhardt, S. (2016). NIH policy on single-IRB review—anew era in multicenter studies. *The New England Journal of Medicine,* 375(24), 2315.

Fålun, N., Fridlund, B., Schaufel, M. A., Schei, E., & Norekvål, T. M. (2016). Patients'goals, resources, and barriers to future change: A qualitative study of patient reflections at hospital discharge after myocardial infarction. *European Journal of Cardiovascular Nursing,* 15(7), 495-503.

Flagg, A. J. (2015). The role of patient-centered care in nursing. *Nursing Clinics,* 50(1), 75-86.

Foster, M. (2015). A new model: the family and child centered care model. *Nursing Praxis in New Zealand,* 31(3), 4.

Fusch, P. I., & Ness, L. R. (2015). Are we there yet? Data saturation in qualitative research. *The Qualitative Report*, 20(9), 1408.

Godin, J., Keefe, J., Kelloway, E. K., & Hirdes, J. P. (2015). Nursing home resident quality of life: testing for measurement equivalence across resident, family, and staff perspectives. *Quality of Life Research*, 24(10), 2365-2374.

Gray, M., Shadden, B., Henry, J., Di Brezzo, R., Ferguson, A., & Fort, I. (2016). Meaning making in long-term care: what do certified nursing assistants think. *Nursing Inquiry,* 23(3), 244-252.

Grosch, K., Medvene, L., & Wolcott, H. (2008). Person-centered caregiving instruction for geriatric nursing assistant students: development and evaluation. *Journal of Gerontological Nursing,* 34(8), 23-31.

Grove, S. K., Burns, N., & Gray, J. (2014). Understanding nursing research: Building anevidence-based practice. Elsevier Health Sciences.

Guest, G., Namey, E., Taylor, J., Eley, N., & McKenna, K. (2017). Comparing focus groups and individual interviews: findings from a randomized study. *International Journal of Social Research Methodology,* 20(6), 693-708.

Halifax, E., Miaskowski, C., & Wallhagen, M. (2018). Certified Nursing Assistants' Understanding of Nursing Home Residents' Pain. *Journal of Gerontological nursing,* 44(4), 29-36.

Hoover, S. M., & Morrow, S. L. (2015). Qualitative researcher reflexivity: A follow-up study with female sexual assault survivors. *The Qualitative Report*, 20(9), 1476.

Hunter, P. V., Hadjistavropoulos, T., & Kaasalainen, S. (2016). A qualitative study of nursing assistants' awareness of person-centered approaches to dementia care. *Ageing & Society,* 36(6), 1211-1237.

Keeley, P., Wolf, Z., Regul, L., & Jadwin, A. (2015). Effectiveness of Standard of Care Protocol on Patient Satisfaction and Perceived Staff Caring. *Clinical Journal of Oncology Nursing,* 19(3), 352-360.

Kehyayan, V., Hirdes, J. P., Tyas, S. L., & Stolee, P. (2015). Residents' self-reported quality of life in long-term care facilities in Canada. *Canadian Journal on Aging/La Revue canadienne du vieillissement,* 34(2), 149- 164.

Kennedy, A., Rogers A., Bowen, R., Lee, V., Blakeman, T., Gardner, C., Morris, R.,…Chew-Graham, C. (2014). Implementing, embedding and integrating self-management support tools for people with long-term conditions in primary care nursing: a qualitative study. *International Journal of Nursing Studies 51, 1103–1113.*

Klapwijk, M. S., Caljouw, M. A., Pieper, M. J., van der Steen, J. T., & Achterberg, W. P. (2016). Characteristics Associated with Quality of Life in Long-Term Care Residents with Dementia: A Cross-Sectional Study. *Dementia and Geriatric Cognitive Disorders,* 42(3-4), 186-197.

Kusmaul, N., & Waldrop, D. P. (2015). Certified nursing assistants as frontline caregivers in nursing homes: Does trauma influence caregiving abilities. *Traumatology,* 21(3), 251.

Kai-Wen, C. (2014). A study on applying focus group interview on education. *Reading Improvement,* 51(4), 381-384.

Labrague, L. J., McEnroe-Petitte, D. M., Papathanasiou, I. V., Edet, O. B., & Arulappan, J. (2015). Impact of instructors' caring on students' perceptions of their own caring behaviors. *Journal of Nursing Scholarship,* 47(4), 338-346.

Lancaster, K. (2017). Confidentiality, anonymity and power relations in elite interviewing: conducting qualitative policy research in a politicised domain. *International Journal of Social Research Methodology*, 20(1), 93-103.

Law, K., Patterson, T. G., & Muers, J. (2017). Staff factors contributing to family satisfaction with long-term dementia care: A systematic review of the literature. *Clinical Gerontologist*, 40(5), 326-351.

Leung, L. (2015). Validity, reliability, and generalizability in qualitative research. *Journal of family medicine and primary care*, 4(3), 324.

Leviton, L. C. (2017). Generalizing about public health interventions: A mixed- methods approach to external validity. *Annual review of public health*, 38, 371-391.

Lewis, S. (2015). Qualitative inquiry and research design: Choosing among five approaches. *Health Promotion Practice*, 16(4), 473-475.

Linzer, M., Poplau, S., Grossman, E., Varkey, A., Yale, S., Williams, E. ... & Barbouche, M. (2015). A cluster randomized trial of interventions to improve work conditions and clinician burnout in primary care: results from the Healthy Work Place (HWP) study. *Journal of General Internal Medicine*, 30(8), 1105-1111.

Lloyd, H., Wheat, H., Horrell, J., Sugavanam, T., Fosh, B., Valderas, J. M., & Close, J. (2018). Patient-reported measures for person-centered coordinated care: a comparative domain map and web-based compendium for supporting policy development and implementation. *Journal of medical Internet research, 20(2).*

Maher, D. (2017). The nursing role in postoperative care of neonates: A qualitative literature review. (Unpublished bachelor thesis). Novia University of Applied Science, Finland.

Martínez, T., Suárez-Álvarez, J., & Yanguas, J. (2016). Instruments for assessing person centered care in gerontology. *Psicothema, 28*(2), 114-121.

McGilton, K. S., Boscart, V. M., Brown, M., & Bowers, B. (2014). Making tradeoffs between the reasons to leave and reasons to stay employed in long-term care homes: Perspectives of licensed nursing staff. *International Journal of Nursing Studies, 51*(6), 917-926.

Noble, H., & Smith, J. (2015). Issues of validity and reliability in qualitative research. *Evidence Based Nursing, 18*(2), 34.

Onwuegbuzie, A. J., Dickinson, W. B., Leech, N. L., & Zoran, A. G. (2009). A qualitative framework for collecting and analyzing data in focus group research. *International Journal of Qualitative methods,* 8(3), 1-21.

O'rourke, H. M., Fraser, K. D., & Duggleby, W. (2015). Does the quality of life construct as illustrated in quantitative measurement tools reflect the perspective of people with dementia. *Journal of Advanced Nursing,* 71(8), 1812-1824.

Rauf, A., Baig, L., Jaffery, T., & Shafi, R. (2014). Exploring the trustworthiness and reliability of focus groups for obtaining useful feedback for evaluation of academic programs. *Education for Health,* 27(1), 28.

Roberts, G., Morley, C., Walters, W., Malta, S., & Doyle, C. (2015). Caring for people with dementia in residential aged care: successes with a composite person-centered care model featuring Montessori-based activities. *Geriatric Nursing,* 36(2), 106-110.

Rodríguez-Martín, B., Stolt, M., Katajisto, J., & Suhonen, R. (2015). Nurses' characteristics and organizational factors associated with their assessments of individualized care in care institutions for older people. *Scandinavian Journal of Caring Sciences, 30(2),* 250-259.

Røen, I., Kirkevold, O., Testad, I., Selbæk, G., Engedal, K., & Bergh, S. (2017). Person centered care in Norwegian nursing homes and its relation to organizational factors and staff characteristics: a cross-sectional survey. *International Psychogeriatrics, 1(12)*.

Ross, H., Tod, A. M., & Clarke, A. (2015). Understanding and achieving person- centered care: the nurse perspective. *Journal of Clinical Nursing, 24(9- 10), 1223-1233.*

Rossi, M. C., Lucisano, G., Funnell, M., Pintaudi, B., Bulotta, A., Gentile, S., .. & BENCH-D Study Group. (2015). Interplay among patient empowerment and clinical and person-centered outcomes in type 2 diabetes. The BENCH-D study. *Patient Education and Counseling,* 98(9), 1142-1149.

Roulston, K., & Shelton, S. A. (2015). Reconceptualizing bias in teaching qualitative research methods. *Qualitative Inquiry, 21(4), 332-342.*

Sanjari, M., Bahramnezhad, F., Fomani, F. K., Shoghi, M., & Cheraghi, M. A. (2014).Ethical challenges of researchers in qualitative studies: the necessity to develop a specific guideline.

Journal of Medical Ethics and History of Medicine, 7, 14.

Seiger C. B., Ternestedt, B. M., & Norberg, A. (2017). Being a close family member of a person with dementia living in a nursing home. *Journal of clinical nursing, 26*(21-22), 3519-3528.

Simmons, S. F., Durkin, D. W., Rahman, A. N., Schnelle, J. F., & Beuscher, L. M. (2014). The value of resident choice during daily care: do staff and families differ. *Journal of Applied Gerontology, 33(6),* 655-671.

Sitzman, K., & Watson, J. (2014). Caring science mindful practice; Implementing Watson's human caring theories. New York, NY: Springer.

Sitzman, K., & Watson, J. (2018). Caring science, mindful practice: Implementing Watson's human caring theory. Springer Publishing Company.

Song, Y., Scales, K., Anderson, R. A., Wu, B., & Corazzini, K. N. (2018). Resident challenges with daily life in Chinese long-term care facilities: A qualitative pilot study. *Geriatric Nursing, 39*(1), 18-23.

Sullivan, J. L., Engle, R. L., Tyler, D., Afable, M. K., Gormley, K.,

Shwartz, M. ... & Parker, V. A. (2018). Is Variation in Resident-Centered Care and Quality Performance Related to Health System Factors in Veterans Health Administration Nursing Homes. INQUIRY: *The Journal of Health Care Organization, Provision, and Financing, 55.*

Tadajewski, M. (2016). Focus groups: history, epistemology and non-individualistic consumer research. *Consumption Markets & Culture,* 19(4), 319-345.

Tayab, A., & Narushima, M. (2014). "Here for the Residents" A Case Study of Cultural Competence of Personal Support Workers in a Long-Term Care Home. *Journal of Transcultural Nursing,* 26(2), 146-156.

Tobiano, G., Bucknall, T., Marshall, A., Guinane, J., & Chaboyer, W. (2015). Nurses' views of patient participation in nursing care. *Journal of Advanced Nursing,* 71(12), 2741-2752.

Tolhurst, E., & Weicht, B. (2017). Preserving personhood: The strategies of men negotiating the experience of dementia. *Journal of Aging Studies,* 40, 29-35.

Turkel, M. C., Watson, J., & Giovannoni, J. (2018). Caring Science or Science of Caring. *Nursing Science Quarterly,* 31(1), 66-71.

Ulin, K., Olsson, L. E., Wolf, A., & Ekman, I. (2016). Person-centered care–An approach that improves the discharge process. *European Journal of Cardiovascular Nursing,* 15(3), 19-e26.

United States Department of Health and Human Services, Centers for Medicare and Medicaid Services. (2017). Transmittal 169—Advance Copy State Operations Manual. Appendix PP–Guidance to surveyors for long-term care facilities. Issued June 30, 2017 (updates current Appendix PP Rev. 168, with phase 2 revisions that become effective 11-28-17)

Van Haitsma, K., Crespy, S., Humes, S., Elliot, A., Mihelic, A., Scott, C. ... Heid, A.R. (2014). New toolkit to measure quality of person-centered care: Development and pilot evaluation with nursing home communities. *Journal of the American Medical Directors Association, 15(9),* 671-680.

Van Hooft S.M., Dwarswaard J., Jedeloo S., Bal R. & van Staa A. (2015). Four perspectives on self-management support by nurses for people with chronic conditions: a Q-methodological study. *International Journal of Nursing Studies* 52, 157–66.

Watson, J., & Brewer, B. B. (2015). Caring science research: Criteria, evidence, and measurement. *Journal of Nursing Administration,*

45(5), 235-236.

Wexler, R., Gerstein, B. S., Brackett, C., Fagnan, L. J. L., Fairfield, K. M., Frosch, D. L., ... & Chang, Y. (2015). Decision Aids in the United States: the Patient Response. *International Journal of Person Centered Medicine*, 5(3), 105-111.

Williams, J., Hadjistavropoulos, T., Ghandehari, O. O., Yao, X., & Lix, L. (2015). An evaluation of a person-centered care programme for long-term care facilities. *Ageing & Society*, 35(3), 457-488.

Wilberforce, M., Challis, D., Davies, L., Kelly, M. P., Roberts, C., & Loynes, N. (2016). Person-centeredness in the care of older adults: a systematic review of questionnaire-based scales and their measurement properties. *BMC Geriatrics*, 16(1), 63.

Wilson, J. (2016). VII—Internal and External Validity in Thought Experiments. In *Proceedings of the Aristotelian Society,* 116(2), 127-152.

Appendix A: Invitation to Participate

Invitation to participate in the research project titled: "Person-centered Care: Perception of the Nurse and Certified Nursing Assistant"

Dear Nurses and Certified Nursing Assistants,

I am conducting focus groups as part of a research study to increase my understanding of how Nurses and Certified Nursing Assistants (CNA) perceive person-centered care. As a nurse/CNA working in a long-term care facility, you are in an ideal position to provide valuable firsthand information from your own perspective.

The focus group discussions will take around 90 minutes and is very informal. I am simply trying to capture your thoughts and perspectives on person-centered care in a long-term care environment. Your responses to the questions will be kept confidential. Each participant will be assigned a number code to help ensure that personal identifiers are not revealed during the analysis and write up of findings. There is no compensation for participating in this study.
However as to the wider community benefits, this study may have a potential social implication of impacting the delivery of care within long-term care settings.

If you are willing to participate please provide your name and contact information to the facility Administrator or Director of Nursing. If you have any questions please do not hesitate to ask.
Thank you for your consideration.

Sincerely,

Appendix B: Focus Group Discussion Script

Moderator Introduction and Purpose (5 minutes):
Welcome and thank you for being here today. My name is LaTonya Hughes and I will conduct the group discussion. The purpose of this gathering is to get your feedback about person-centered care. There are no right or wrong answers. Your personal opinions and views are very important. The discussion will last for about one hour. I ask you to please switch off your mobile phones. Any questions? Let's now discuss how the group discussion will be held.

Procedure (5 minutes):
I will guide the conversation by asking questions pertaining to person-centered care. This conversation will be recorded. The recording will only be used to make sure my notes are correct. I will be the only person listening to the tape. This is a confidential discussion in that I will not report who or what is said to your colleagues or supervisors. No names or personal information will be used in the report.

Ground Rules (5 minutes):
I ask that you please give everyone the chance to express their opinion during the conversation. Only one person speaks at a time. It may be difficult to capture everyone's experience and perspective on the audio recording if there are multiple voices at once. Any questions?

Introduction of Participants (15 minutes):
Before we get started, I'd like to know a little about each of you. Please tell me your name, your role and why do you like working in long-term care (engagement question).

Nice to meet you all. Now we have introduced ourselves, let us move right into our focus group questions:

Theoretical Framework Discussion
Jean Watson's caring theory is the theoretical framework used for this study. Jean Watson believes that 10 factors are associated with caring. Here is a list of the 10 factors. As you answer the research questions, you are welcome to take these factors into consideration.

Focus Group Questions (55 minutes):
1. Tell me about the care residents received here.
2. What is your understanding of person-centered care?
3. How do you know that you have provided person-centered care?

Closing (5 minutes):
Thank you for participating today. Is there anything else you would like to say about person-centered care (exit question)? Your comments have given me lots of insight. I thank you for your time

www.ingramcontent.com/pod-product-compliance
Lightning Source LLC
Chambersburg PA
CBHW021446210526
45463CB00002B/656